A Springs
Book

IN PRAISE
OF BEAUTY

GW00706185

Shakespeare

Search Press Ltd, England
Kampmann & Company Inc, New York

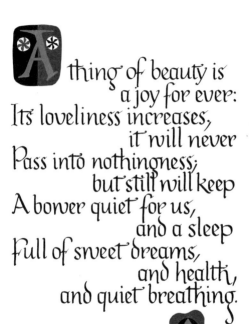

A thing of beauty is
        a joy for ever:
Its loveliness increases,
        it will never
Pass into nothingness;
        but still will keep
A bower quiet for us,
        and a sleep
Full of sweet dreams,
        and health,
    and quiet breathing.

KEATS

Beauty
is a rare
miracle
that reduces
to silence
our doubts
about God.

JEAN ANOUILH

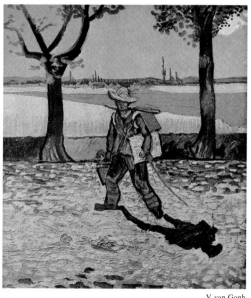

V. van Gogh

With hue like that when some great painter drops
His pencil in the gloom of earthquake and eclipse.

SHELLEY

The most beautiful
thing that we can
experience is
            mystery.
He who does not
know it, and does
not marvel at it, is,
one might say,
dead and his
            vision extinct.

 ALBERT EINSTEIN

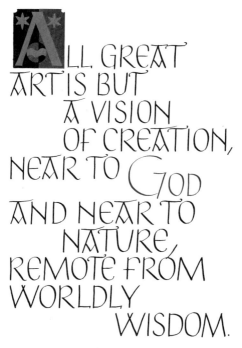

ALL GREAT
ART IS BUT
A VISION
OF CREATION,
NEAR TO GOD
AND NEAR TO
NATURE,
REMOTE FROM
WORLDLY
WISDOM.

MANFRED KYBER

The painter creates with brush and palette something which gives as much pleasure to the eye as music does to the ear.

LEONARDO DA VINCI

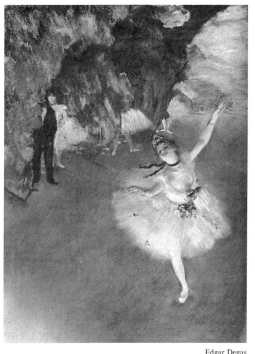

Edgar Degas

He who has the ability to perceive beauty never
grows old.   FRANZ KAFKA

Not only philosophy, but art and beauty combine to solve the mystery of life.

ARTHUR SCHOPENHAUER

Beauty and perfection change and are transformed continually. Only what is simple and natural defies change.

G. SEGANTINI

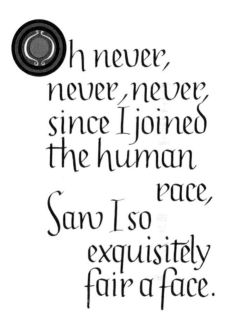

Oh never,
never, never,
since I joined
the human
                race,
Saw I so
        exquisitely
        fair a face.

W·S·GILBERT

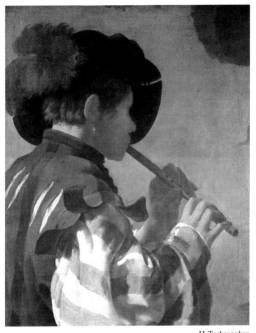

H. Terbrugghen

Art is not the bread, but the wine of life.

JEAN PAUL.

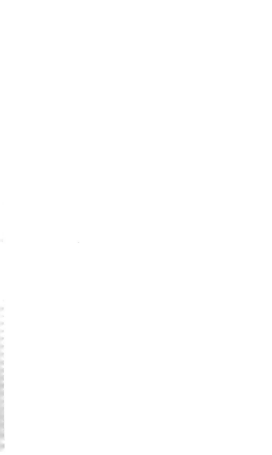

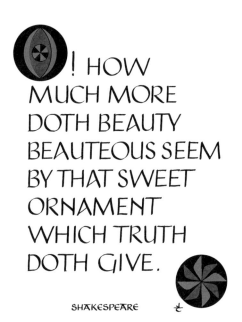

O! HOW MUCH MORE DOTH BEAUTY BEAUTEOUS SEEM BY THAT SWEET ORNAMENT WHICH TRUTH DOTH GIVE.

SHAKESPEARE

What comes to
perfection perishes.
Things learned
on earth we
shall practise
in heaven.
Works done
least rapidly,
Art most
cherishes.

BROWNING

True ease in
writing comes
from art, not
           chance,
As those who
move easiest
who have
learned
          to dance.

ALEXANDER POPE

Beauty

is

altogether

in the

eye of

the

beholder.

LEW WALLACE

Orpheus with his lute
        made trees,
And the mountain-tops
        that freeze,
Bow themselves when
        he did sing:
To his music plants
        and flowers
Ever sprung, as sun
        and showers
There had made a
        lasting spring.

SHAKESPEARE

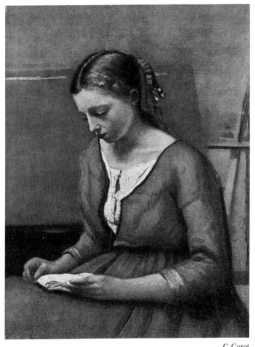

C. Corot

Beauty in things exists in the mind which
contemplates them.   DAVID HUME

Beauty is
truth,
truth beauty –
that is all
Ye know on earth,
and all ye
need to know.

KEATS

Precious little gifts of lasting value

In the same series:

Springs of Joy	Springs of Chinese Wisdom
Springs of Humor	Springs of Hope
Springs of Oriental Wisdom	Springs of Happiness
Springs of Greek Wisdom	Springs of Animal Wisdom
Springs of Indian Wisdom	Spirit of American Wit
Springs of Love	Springs of Comfort
Springs of Roman Wisdom	Springs of Russian Wisdom
Springs of Consolation	Springs of Japanese Wisdom
Springs of Jewish Wisdom	Springs of Islamic Wisdom
Springs of Friendship	Springs of Music
Springs of African Wisdom	Springs of Peace
Springs of Persian Wisdom	Affection, Friendship and Love

Text chosen by Eugen Hettinger
Graphic presentation: Josef Tannheimer
Translator: Charlotte de la Bedoyère

Cover picture: Botticelli, Birth of Venus (detail)
Reprinted by kind permission of the publishers

Distribution: Search Press Ltd., England

Copyright 1984 by Leobuchhandlung, CH-St.Gallen
Modèle déposé, BIRPI
Printed in Switzerland